Student Nurse Planner

All the Tools You Need to Be Successful in Nursing School!

Dear Student,

My name is T.L. Campbell, M.S.N. R.N. and I have been a Registered Nurse for the past 10 years. I currently serve as the Vice President of Clinical Operations and Quality Excellence for A healthcare company in Texas.

As you begin your long and challenging journey to becoming a nurse, you will find that you will need to be very organized. You will have more books and papers than you'll know what to do with and you will need to access certain information very quickly.

I compiled this book just for that purpose. Please keep it close so that you'll be able to use it freely.

One thing all nursing students are asked to do is to keep a journal of your thoughts and experiences. Some Nursing Instructors may even ask to see it. I have included many pages for you to journal on throughout your student experience.

You will find quick references for lab values and conversions here as well. And if you don't know Spanish, never fear, as a bonus I put quite a few Spanish phrases that helped me with the Spanish-speaking patient population.

My hope is that you will find this book different than any other on the market. First, it has been created by a genuine R.N., who knows what it's like to survive, yes survive, Nursing School. So, I've put a few goodies in the book that I really needed all in one spot throughout my classes and clinicals.

Second, this book is far more than just a journal; it is a functional toolbox for you to utilize which includes:

- Emergency Contact List
- Lab Values Quick Reference Guide
- Spanish Phrases for Student Nurses
- Self-dateable Clinical Planning Calendar
- Conversion Table

As you use it, you will see the arc you have taken from your first day of school to your graduation ceremony.

Best of luck to you,

Trace Campbell, M.S.N., R.N.

Vice President of Clinical Operations

and Quality Excellence

EMERGENCY CONTACT LIST

LOCAL CONTACT

Name

Phone

Alternate Phone

OUT OF STATE CONTACT

Name

Phone

Alternate Phone

NEXT OF KIN

Name

Phone

Alternate Phone

WORK CONTACT

Name

Phone

Alternate Phone

PHYSICIAN NAME

Name

Phone

Alternate Phone

NEIGHBOR/LANLORD/ HOMEWONER ASSOCIATION

Name

Phone

Alternate Phone

EMERGENCY SERVICES

Police/Ambulance: 911

Fire Department:

Poison Control:

LOCAL SERVICES

Gas Company:

Electric Company:

Water Company:

OTHER EMERGENCY CONTACTS

Name

Phone

Alternate Phone

OTHER EMERGENCY CONTACTS

Name

Phone

Alternate Phone

CONTACT LIST

Name	Ph. Number	Email	Company

Conversion Table

1 milliliter (mL)	=1 cubic centimeter (cc)
1 teaspoon (tsp)	= 5 milliliters (mL)
1000 milliliters (mL)	= 1 Liter (L)
3 teaspoon (tsp)	= 1 tablespoon (Tbsp)
1000 micrograms (mcg)	= 1 milligram (mg)
2 tablespoons (Tbsp)	= 1 ounce (oz)
1000 Grams (G)	= 1 Kilogram (Kg)
30 milliliters (mL)	= 1 ounce (oz)
1000 milligrams (mg)	= 1 Gram (G)
2.2 pounds (lb)	= 1 Kilogram (Kg)
1 tablespoon (Tbsp)	= 15 milliliters (ml)

Spanish Phrases for the Student Nurse

Introduction phrases:

Hello, my name is _____ and I'll be your nurse
Hola, me llamo _____ y soy su enfermera (o).

What is your name?
Como se llama?

How old are you?
Cuántos años tiene usted?

How are you today?
Como esta hoy?

I don't speak Spanish very well.
No hablo español muy bien.

Exam phrases:

Inhale.
Aspire.

Exhale.
Exhále.

Breathe deeply.

Respire profundomente.

Are you in pain?

Tiene dolor?

I am going to take your temperature.

Le voy a tomar su temperatura.

Don't throw away urine/ stool.

No tire la orina / popo.

Do you feel lightheaded/ dizzy?

Se siente mareado?

Are you pregnant?

Está embarazada?

Have you been in the hospital before?

Ha estado en el hospital antes?

What medicines are your allergic to? (a) None (b) Penicillin (c) Tetanus (d) Sulfas (e) Aspirin

A qué medicinas tiene usted alergia? (a) A ninguna (b) A la penicilina (c) A la vacuna contra el tétano (d) A las sulfas (e) la aspirina

What medicines do you take?

Qué medicinas toma?

Where does it hurt? Here?
Dónde le duele? Aqui?

Is it constant pain or does it come and go?
Es un dolor constante o viene y se va?

How long have you had it?
Désde cuándo lo tiene?

Has the pain increased or decreased?
Ha aumentado o disminuído el dolor?

Cough!
Tosa!

Misc. phrases:

Speak slowly, please.
Hable despacio por favor.

Repeat, please
Repita, por favor.

I don't understand.
No entiendo.

I'll be back in a moment.
Regreso en un momento.

Permit me.
Permítame.

Relax.
Ud. relájase.

Use the call light if you need help.
Use el botón para ayuda.

Ask for help before you get up.
Llame antes de levantarse.

Do you want to use the restroom?
Quiere ir al baño?

Do you want to take a shower?
Quiere bañarse?

I am going to give you an injection.
Le voy a poner una inyección.

I am going to place an intravenous needle in your arm.
Le voy a poner una agúja intravenosa en el brazo.

Do you have questions?
Tienes preguntas?

Value	Normal Range	Unit
COMPLETE BLOOD COUNT		
Red Blood Cell (RBC)	M: 4.5 - 5.5 F: 4.0 - 4.9	x10 5 /ml
White Blood Cell (WBC)	4,500 - 10,000	cells/mcL
Platelets	100,000 - 450, 000	cells/mcL
Hemoglobin (Hgb)	M: 13.5 - 16.5 F: 12.0 - 15.0 Preg: 10 - 15	g/dL
Hematocrit (Hct)	M: 41 - 50% F: 36 - 44%	N/A
Mean Corpuscular Vol. (MCV)	80 - 100	fL

DIFFERENTIAL COUNT		
Neutrophils	54 - 62%	N/A
Eosinophils	1 - 3%	N/A
Basophils	0 - 0.75%	N/A
Lymphocytes	25 - 33%	N/A
Monocytes	3 - 7%	N/A

SERUM ELECTROLYTES		
Sodium (Na+)	135 - 145	mEq/L
Potassium (K+)	3.5 - 5.5	mEq/L
Chloride (Cl-)	95 - 105	mEq/L
Calcium	8.5 - 10.9	mEq/L
Calcium (ionized)	2.24 - 2.46	mEq/L
Magnesium (Mg)	1.5 - 2.5	mEq/L
Phosphorus (P)	2.5 - 4.5	mEq/L

URINALYSIS		
Volume	1,000 - 2,000	mL/day
	30	mL/hour
Specific Gravity	1.010 - 1.020	N/A
pH	4.5 - 8	N/A
Casts	1 - 2	per field
Glucose	none	N/A
Protein	none	N/A
Uric Acid	M: 2.6 - 6.0 F: 3.5 - 7.2	mg/dL

Value	Normal Range	Unit
CHEMISTRY VALUES		
Adult Glucose	70 - 110	mg/dL
Blood Urea Nitrogen (BUN)	Adult 7 – 18 Pedi 5 – 20 Infant 5 - 15	mg/dL
Serum Creatinine	0.6 - 1.35	mg/dL
Creatine phosphokinase (CPK)	21 - 198	units/L
Creatinine Clearance (CrCl)	M: 90 - 138 F: 85 - 132	mL/min
Albumin	3.4 - 5.0	g/dL
Bilirubin	< 1.0	mg/dL
Uric Acid	3.5 - 7.5	mg/dL

COAGULATION STUDIES		
Prothrombin Time (PT)	11 - 14	seconds
Partial Thromboplastin Time (PTT)	25 - 35	seconds
International Normalized Ratio (INR)	0.8 -1.2	N/A
Activated Partial Thromboplastin Time (aPTT)	1.5 - 2.5	N/A
Fibrinogen	203 - 377	mg/dL
Bleeding time	1 - 6	Mins.

LIPOPROTEINS AND TRIGLYCERIDES		
Total Cholesterol	Ideal: below 200 Borderline: 200 - 240 High: above 240	mg/dL
Low Density Lipoprotein (LDL)	< 70	mg/dL
High Density Lipoprotein (HDL)	< 60	mg/dL
Triglycerides	Normal: below 150 Borderline high: 150 - 199 High: 200 - 499 Very high: above 500	mg/dL
SGOT (AST)	< 35	IU/L
SGPT (ALT)	< 35	IU/L

Value	Normal Range	Unit
CARDIAC MARKERS		
Troponin (CTN-1 or CTN-T)	Normal I: 0.03 Critical level I: above 1.5 Critical level T: 0.2	ng/L
C-reactive protein	Below 0.8	mg/dL
CD40 Ligand	1.51 - 5.35	mg/L
Creatinine Kinase (CK-MB)	0 - 3	mcg/L

ARTERIAL BLOOD GASSES		
pH	7.35 - 7.45	N/A
Partial Pressure of CO_2 (pCO_2)	35—45	mmHg
Partial Pressure of O_2 (pO_2)	80 - 100	mmHg
Bicarbonate (HCO_3)	22 - 26	mEq/L
Base Excess (BE)	-2 to +2	mEq/L
Oxygen Saturation (SaO_2)	95 - 100%	N/A

THYROID FUNCTION STUDIES		
Thyroid-Stimulating Hormone (TSH)	Adults: 0.2 - 5.4 Neonate: 3 - 20	mU/L
Thyroxine (Total T_4)	Adult: 5.4 - 11.5 Child: 6.4 - 13.3	mcg/dL
Free Thyroxine (Total T_4 F $_4$)	Adult: 0.7 - 2.0	ng/dL

CLASS AND CLINICALS SCHEDULE: ___ / ___ /20___

Sunday	Monday	Tuesday	Wednesday	Thursday	Friday	Saturday

CLASS AND CLINICALS SCHEDULE:

___/___/20___

Sunday	Monday	Tuesday	Wednesday	Thursday	Friday	Saturday

CLASS AND CLINICALS SCHEDULE:

____ / ____ /20____

Sunday	Monday	Tuesday	Wednesday	Thursday	Friday	Saturday

CLASS AND CLINICALS SCHEDULE:

___/____/20___

Sunday	Monday	Tuesday	Wednesday	Thursday	Friday	Saturday

CLASS AND CLINICALS SCHEDULE:

_____ / _____ /20_____

Sunday	Monday	Tuesday	Wednesday	Thursday	Friday	Saturday

CLASS AND CLINICALS SCHEDULE:

_____ / _____ /20_____

Sunday	Monday	Tuesday	Wednesday	Thursday	Friday	Saturday

CLASS AND CLINICALS SCHEDULE:

_____ / _____ /20_____

Sunday	Monday	Tuesday	Wednesday	Thursday	Friday	Saturday

CLASS AND CLINICALS SCHEDULE:

_____ / _____ /20_____

Sunday	Monday	Tuesday	Wednesday	Thursday	Friday	Saturday

CLASS AND CLINICALS SCHEDULE:

_____/_____/20_____

Sunday	Monday	Tuesday	Wednesday	Thursday	Friday	Saturday

CLASS AND CLINICALS SCHEDULE:

____ / ____ /20____

Sunday	Monday	Tuesday	Wednesday	Thursday	Friday	Saturday

CLASS AND CLINICALS SCHEDULE:

_____ / _____ /20_____

Sunday	Monday	Tuesday	Wednesday	Thursday	Friday	Saturday